MedicalCenter.com

The Key Facts on Breast Cancer

I0470642

Everything You Need to Know About Breast Cancer

By Patrick W. Nee

www.MedicalCenter.com

Published by:

MedicalCenter.com

96 Walter Street/ Suite 200

Boston, MA 02131, USA

Tel: 617-354-7722

www.MedicalCenter.com

manager@medicalcenter.com

Table of Contents

Chapter 1: What is Breast Cancer?

How Tumors Form

The body is made up of many types of cells. Normally, cells grow, divide and produce more cells as needed to keep the body healthy. Sometimes, however, the process goes wrong. Cells become abnormal and form more cells in an uncontrolled way. These extra cells form a mass of tissue, called a growth or tumor. Tumors can be benign, which means not cancerous, or malignant, which means cancerous. Breast cancer occurs when malignant tumors form in the breast tissue.

Who Gets Breast Cancer?

Breast cancer is one of the most common cancers in American women. It is more common among older women than younger women. Men can get breast cancer too, although they account for only one percent of all reported cases.

When Breast Cancer Spreads

When cancer grows in breast tissue and spreads outside the breast, cancer cells are often found in the lymph nodes under the arm. If the cancer has reached these nodes, it means that cancer cells may have spread, or metastasized, to other parts of the body.

When cancer spreads from its original location in the breast to another part of the body such as the brain, it is called metastatic breast cancer, not brain cancer. Doctors sometimes call this "distant" disease.

Breast Cancer is Not Contagious

Breast cancer is not contagious. A woman cannot "catch" breast cancer from other women who have the disease. Also, breast cancer is not caused by an injury to the breast. Most women who develop breast cancer do not have any known risk factors or a history of the disease in their families.

Treating and Surviving Breast Cancer

Today, more women are surviving breast cancer than ever before. Over two million women are breast cancer survivors. There are several ways to treat breast cancer, but all treatments work best when the disease is found early. As a matter of fact, when it is caught in its earliest stage, 98 percent of women with the disease are alive five years later. Every day researchers are working to find new and better ways to detect and treat cancer. Many studies of new approaches for women with breast cancer are under way. With early detection, and prompt and appropriate treatment, the outlook for women with breast cancer can be positive.

Chapter 2: Risk Factors

No one knows why some women develop breast cancer and others do not. Although the disease may affect younger women, three-fourths of all breast cancers occur in women age 50 or older.

In Situ and Invasive Breast Cancer

Researchers often talk about breast cancer in two ways: *in situ* and invasive. *In situ* refers to cancer that has not spread beyond its site of origin. Invasive applies to cancer that has spread to the tissue around it.

This chart shows what the approximate chances are of a woman getting invasive breast cancer in her lifetime.

Ages	Chances
30 to 40...	Chances are 1 out of 227
40 to 50...	Chances are 1 out of 68
50 to 60...	Chances are 1 out of 41
60 to 70...	Chances are 1 out of 27
70 to 80...	Chances are 1 out of 25

Risk Factors

Older age and the following risk factors increase a woman's chance of getting breast cancer. Risk factors are conditions or agents that increase a person's chances of getting a disease.

- Breast cancer among one or more of your close relatives, such as a sister, mother, or daughter.
- Having no children or having your first child in your mid-thirties or later.
- Having your first menstrual period before age 12.
- Gaining weight after menopause, especially after natural menopause and/or after age 60.
- Race. White women are at greater risk than black women. However, black women diagnosed with breast cancer are more likely to die of the disease.

Five percent to 10 percent of all breast cancers are thought to be inherited.

Warning Signs

When breast cancer first develops, there may be no symptoms at all. But as the cancer grows, it can cause changes that women should watch for. You can help safeguard your health by learning the following warning signs of breast cancer.

- A lump or thickening in or near the breast or in the underarm area.
- A change in the size or shape of the breast.
- Nipple discharge or tenderness, or the nipple is pulled back or inverted into the breast.
- Ridges or pitting of the breast. The skin looks like the skin of an orange.
- A change in the way the skin of the breast, areola, or nipple looks or feels. For example, the skin may be warm, swollen, red, or scaly.

Don't Ignore Symptoms

You should see your doctor about any symptoms like these. Most often, they are not cancer, but it's important to check with the doctor so that any problems can be diagnosed and treated as early as possible.

Some women believe that as they age, health problems are due to "growing older." Because of this myth, many illnesses go undiagnosed and untreated. Don't ignore your symptoms because you think they are not important or because you believe they are normal for your age. Talk to your doctor.

Chapter 3: Tests and Diagnosis

Most cancers in their early, most treatable stages do not cause any symptoms. That is why it's important to have regular tests to check for cancer long before you might notice anything wrong.

Detecting Breast Cancer Through Screening

When breast cancer is found early, it is more likely to be treated successfully. Checking for cancer in a person who does not have any symptoms is called screening. Screening tests for breast cancer include, among others, clinical breast exams and mammograms. Recent studies have shown that ultrasound and MRI's may also be useful complementary screening tools, particularly in women with mammograms that are not definitive.

During a clinical breast exam, the doctor or other health care professional checks the breasts and underarms for lumps or other changes that could be a sign of breast cancer. A mammogram is a special x-ray of the breast that often can detect cancers that are too small for a woman or her doctor to feel.

Who Should Have a Mammography?

Several studies show that mammography screening has reduced the number of deaths from breast cancer. However, some other studies have not shown a clear benefit from mammography.

Scientists are continuing to examine the level of benefit that mammography can produce. The National Cancer Institute recommends the following:

- If you are a woman in your 40s, you should have mammography screening every one to two years.
- If you are a woman age 50 and older, you should have mammography screening every one to two years.
- If you are a woman who is at higher than average risk for breast cancer, you should seek expert medical advice about whether to begin screening before age 40 and how often to have screening mammography.

Between 5 and 10 percent of mammogram results are abnormal and require more testing. Most of these follow-up tests confirm that no cancer was present.

How Biopsies are Performed

If needed, the most common follow-up test a doctor will recommend is called a biopsy. This is a procedure where a small amount of fluid or tissue is removed from the breast to make a diagnosis. A doctor might perform fine needle aspiration, a needle or core biopsy, or a surgical biopsy.

- **With fine needle aspiration**, doctors numb the area and use a thin needle to remove fluid and/or cells from a breast lump. If the fluid is clear, it may not need to be checked out by a lab.

- **For a needle biopsy**, sometimes called a core biopsy, doctors use a needle to remove tissue from an area that looks suspicious on a mammogram but cannot be felt. This tissue goes to a lab where a pathologist examines it to see if any of the cells are cancerous.

- **In a surgical biopsy**, a surgeon removes a sample of a lump or suspicious area. Sometimes it is necessary to remove the entire lump or suspicious area, plus an area of healthy tissue around the edges. The tissue then goes to a lab where a pathologist examines it under a microscope to check for cancer cells.

Another type of surgical biopsy that removes less breast tissue is called an image-guided needle breast biopsy, or stereotactic biopsy.

Eighty percent of U.S. women who have a surgical breast biopsy do not have cancer. However, women who have breast biopsies are at higher risk of developing breast cancer than women who have never had a breast biopsy.

Other Detection Methods

Magnetic resonance imaging, or MRI, and ultrasound are two other techniques which, as supplements to standard mammography, might help detect breast cancer with greater accuracy.

Genetic Detection

The most comprehensive study to date of gene mutations in breast cancer, published in September 2012, confirmed that there are four primary subtypes of breast cancer, each with its own biology. The four groups are called intrinsic subtypes of breast cancer and include HER2-enriched (HER2E), Luminal A (LumA), Luminal B (LumB) and Basal-like. The outlook for survival is different for each of these subtypes of breast cancer.

Researchers found that one subtype, Basal-like breast cancer, shares many genetic features with a form of ovarian cancer, and that both may respond similarly to drugs that reduce tumor growth or target DNA repair.

The authors hope that discovery of these mutations will be an important step in the effort to improve therapies for breast cancer. For the time being, there are no genetic tests that are commercially available based solely on these findings. Soon, however, knowing extensively which breast cancer gene mutations a woman has should help guide precision treatment.

Chapter 4: Planning Treatment

There are many treatment options for women with breast cancer. The choice of treatment depends on your age and general health, the stage of the cancer, whether or not it has spread beyond the breast, and other factors.

If tests show that you have cancer, you should talk with your doctor and make treatment decisions as soon as possible. Studies show that early treatment leads to better outcomes.

Working With a Team of Specialists

People with cancer often are treated by a team of specialists. The team will keep the primary doctor informed about the patient's progress. The team may include a medical oncologist who is a specialist in cancer treatment, a surgeon, a radiation oncologist who is a specialist in radiation therapy, and others. Before starting treatment, you may want another doctor to review the diagnosis and treatment plan. Some insurance companies require a second opinion. Others may pay for a second opinion if you request it.

Clinical Trials for Breast Cancer

Some breast cancer patients take part in studies of new treatments. These studies, called clinical trials, are designed to find out whether a new treatment is both safe and effective.

Often, clinical trials compare a new treatment with a standard one so that doctors can learn which is more effective. Women with breast cancer who are interested in taking part in a clinical trial should talk to their doctor.

Chapter 5: Staging

What Staging Reveals

Once breast cancer has been found, it is staged. Staging means determining how far the cancer has progressed. Through staging, the doctor can tell if the cancer has spread and, if so, to what parts of the body. More tests may be performed to help determine the stage. Knowing the stage of the disease helps the doctor plan treatment.

Staging will let the doctor know

- the size of the tumor and exactly where it is in the breast
- if the cancer has spread within the breast
- if cancer is present in the lymph nodes under the arm
- if cancer is present in other parts of the body

Stages of Breast Cancer

- **Stage 0** -- This is very early breast cancer that has not spread within or outside the breast. Doctors often refer to this type of cancer as *in situ* or non-invasive cancer.
- **Stage I and stage II** also are early stages of breast cancer. Stage I means that the tumor has not spread beyond the breast. In stage II,

the tumor may be larger and may have spread to the lymph nodes.

- **Stage III** is called locally advanced cancer. Here the tumor has spread beyond the breast to lymph nodes or to other tissues near the breast.
- **Stage IV** is metastatic cancer. In this stage the cancer has spread beyond the breast and the underarm lymph nodes to other parts of the body, most often the bones, lungs, liver, or brain.

The choice of treatment is based on many factors. For stage I, II or III cancers, the main goals are to treat the cancer and reduce the chance it will come back, either at the place where the tumor first occurred or elsewhere in the body. For stage IV cancer, the goal is to improve symptoms and prolong survival.

Chapter 6: Standard Treatments

There are a number of treatments for breast cancer, but the ones women choose most often -- alone or in combination -- are surgery, radiation therapy, chemotherapy, and hormone therapy.

What Standard Treatments Do

Here is what the standard cancer treatments are designed to do:

- **Surgery** takes out the cancer.
- **Hormone therapy** keeps cancer cells from getting the hormones they need to survive and grow.
- **Radiation therapy** uses high-energy beams to kill cancer cells and shrink tumors.
- **Chemotherapy** uses anti-cancer drugs to kill cancer cells.

Treatment for breast cancer may involve local or whole body therapy. Doctors use local therapies, such as surgery or radiation, to remove or destroy breast cancer in a specific area. Whole body, or systemic, treatments like chemotherapy, hormonal, or biological therapies are used to destroy or control cancer throughout the body. Some patients have both kinds of treatment.

Treating Early-Stage Breast Cancer

If you have early-stage breast cancer, one common treatment available to you is a lumpectomy combined with radiation therapy. A lumpectomy is surgery that preserves a woman's breast.

In a lumpectomy, the surgeon removes only the tumor and a small amount of the surrounding tissue. The survival rate for a woman who has this therapy plus radiation is similar to that for a woman who chooses a radical mastectomy, which is complete removal of a breast.

If Cancer Has Spread Locally

If you have breast cancer that has spread locally -- just to other parts of the breast -- your treatment may involve a combination of chemotherapy and surgery. Doctors first shrink the tumor with chemotherapy and then remove it through surgery. Shrinking the tumor before surgery may allow a woman to avoid a mastectomy and keep her breast.

In the past, doctors would remove a lot of lymph nodes near breast tumors to see if the cancer had spread. Some doctors also use a method called sentinel node biopsy. Using a dye or radioactive tracer, surgeons locate the first or sentinel lymph node closest to the tumor, and remove only that node to see if the cancer has spread.

If Cancer Has Spread Beyond the Breast

If the breast cancer has spread to other parts of the body, such as the lung or bone, you might receive chemotherapy and/or hormonal therapy to destroy cancer cells and control the disease. Radiation therapy may also be useful to control tumors in other parts of the body.

Chapter 7: Latest Research

New Technologies

Several new technologies offer hope for making future treatment easier for women with breast cancer. Using a special tool, doctors can today insert a miniature camera through the nipple and into a milk duct in the breast to examine the area for cancer.

Researchers are testing another technique to help women who have undergone weeks of conventional radiation therapy. Using a small catheter -- a tube with a balloon tip -- doctors can deliver tiny radioactive beads to a place on the breast where cancer tissue has been removed. This can reduce the therapy time to a matter of days.

New Drug Combination Therapies

New drug therapies and combination therapies continue to evolve.

A mix of drugs may increase the length of time you will live or the length of time you will live without cancer. It may someday prove useful for some women with localized breast cancer after they have had surgery.

New research shows women with early-stage breast cancer who took the drug letrozole, an aromatase inhibitor, after they completed five years of tamoxifen therapy significantly reduced their risk of breast cancer recurrence.

Treating HER2-Positive Breast Cancer

Herceptin® is a drug commonly used to treat women who have a certain type of breast cancer. This drug slows or stops the growth of cancer cells by blocking HER2, a protein found on the surface of some types of breast cancer cells. Approximately 20 to 25 percent of breast cancers produce too much HER2. These "HER2 positive" tumors tend to grow faster and are generally more likely to return than tumors that do not overproduce HER2.

Results from clinical trials show that those patients with early-stage HER2 positive breast cancer who received Herceptin® in combination with chemotherapy had a 52 percent decrease in risk in the cancer returning compared with patients who received chemotherapy treatment alone. Cancer treatments like chemotherapy can be systemic, meaning they affect whole tissues, organs, or the entire body. Herceptin®, however, was the first drug used to target only a specific molecule involved in breast cancer. Another drug, Tykerb®, was approved by the U.S. Food and Drug Administration for use for treatment of HER2-positive breast cancer. Because of the availability of these two drugs, an international trial called ALTTO was designed to determine if one drug is more effective, safer, and if taking the drugs separately, in tandem order, or together is better.

The TAILORx Trial

In an attempt to further specialize breast cancer treatment, The Trial Assigning Individualized Options for Treatment, or TAILORx, enrolled 10,000 women to examine whether appropriate treatment can be assigned based on genes that are frequently associated with risk of recurrence of breast cancer. The goal of TAILORx is important because the majority of women with early-stage breast cancer are advised to receive chemotherapy in addition to radiation and hormonal therapy, yet research has not demonstrated that chemotherapy benefits all of them equally.

TAILORx seeks to examine many of a woman's genes simultaneously and use this information in choosing a treatment course, thus sparing women unnecessary treatment if chemotherapy is not likely to be of substantial benefit to them.

Several methods can reduce the risk of breast cancer. The drug tamoxifen has been proven to lower the chance of cancer in high-risk women.

A clinical trial of this drug sponsored by the National Cancer Institute that included more than 13,000 pre-menopausal and post-menopausal women. All of the women were considered at high risk for breast cancer.

One group of women took the drug tamoxifen and another took a placebo -- an inactive pill that looked like tamoxifen. The results of the study showed a 49 percent decrease in breast cancer among women who took tamoxifen.

Tamoxifen does have side effects. The most serious in some women are an increased risk of endometrial cancer, uterine sarcoma, and an increased risk of blood clots. Women at high risk for breast cancer may want to consult their doctor to see if tamoxifen may help them.

The STAR Trial

The Study of Tamoxifen and Raloxifene (STAR) was another clinical trial sponsored by the National Cancer Institute.

STAR enlisted nearly 20,000 women to compare tamoxifen to the drug raloxifene for effectiveness in reducing of breast cancer risk.

Raloxifene, marketed as Evista®, has been approved for use to lower the risk of and treat osteoporosis.

Results of the STAR trial show that raloxifene works as well as tamoxifen in reducing breast cancer risk for postmenopausal women at increased risk of the disease. Both drugs decrease risk by about 50 percent.

In addition, women enrolled in STAR who were assigned to take raloxifene had fewer uterine cancers, blood clots, and cataracts than those taking tamoxifen.

However, taking raloxifene raised the risk of blood clots and fatal strokes in women already at risk.

Chapter 8: Frequently Asked Questions

1. What is cancer?

The body is made up of many types of cells. Normally, cells grow, divide, and produce more cells as needed to keep the body healthy. Sometimes, however, the process goes wrong. Cells become abnormal and form more cells in an uncontrolled way. These extra cells form a mass of tissue, called a growth or tumor. Tumors can be benign, which means not cancerous, or malignant, which means cancerous.

2. What is breast cancer?

Breast cancer occurs when a malignant tumor forms in the breast tissue. The cancer can be found in the breast itself or in the ducts and lymph nodes that surround the breast.

3. What is metastatic breast cancer?

When cancer spreads from its original location in the breast to another part of the body such as the brain, it is called metastatic breast cancer, not brain cancer. Doctors sometimes call this "distant" disease.

4. Do men get breast cancer?

Yes. Although breast cancer is primarily a woman's disease, men can get breast cancer too. They can develop it at any age, but they are usually between 60 and 70 years of age when the diagnosis is made. Male breast cancer makes up less than 1 percent of all cases of breast cancer.

5. What are the chances of surviving breast cancer?

One definition of cure is being alive and free of breast cancer for 5 years. If the cancer is found early, a woman's chances of survival are better. In fact, nearly 98 percent of women who discover their breast cancer when it is near the site of origin and still small in size are alive 5 years later.

However, women whose cancer is diagnosed at a late stage, after it has spread to other parts of the body, have only a 23.3 percent chance of surviving 5 years.

6. What is the most important risk factor for breast cancer?

Older age is a major risk factor. Three-fourths of all breast cancers occur in women age 50 or older. Having a sister, mother, or daughter who has had breast cancer also increases your risk.

7. What role do gene mutations play in breast cancer?

A full analysis of all of the genes that determine cancer outcomes remains a difficult challenge. However, recent results from The Cancer Genome Atlas, an NIH study that included analyses of gene mutations in breast cancer, provide a list of mutations for other scientists to study and explore.

Many clinical trials now include gene profiles of cancer patients as a way to tell how cancer may progress or be diagnosed. Gene profiles are even used to monitor how cancer genes are affected by targeted therapies. The knowledge from this new study will be used to bring earlier and better treatments to cancer patients.

8. What are the symptoms of breast cancer?

When breast cancer first develops, there may be no symptoms at all. But as the cancer grows, it can cause changes that women should watch for. You can help safeguard your health by learning the following warning signs of breast cancer:

- a lump or thickening in or near the breast or in the underarm area.
- a change in the size or shape of the breast.
- ridges or pitting of the breast; the skin looks like the skin of an orange.
- a change in the way the skin of the breast, areola, or nipple looks or feels; for example, it may be warm, swollen, red, or scaly.
- nipple discharge or tenderness, or the nipple is pulled back or inverted into the breast.

9. Should I perform regular breast self-exams?

Doing a breast self-exam may help a woman detect a lump that might otherwise go unnoticed. However, most health organizations currently recommend clinical breast exams done by a doctor or trained expert, or mammograms, as the most reliable tools for detecting breast cancer.

10. What happens during a clinical breast exam?

During a clinical breast exam, a doctor or other health care professional checks the breasts and underarms for lumps or other changes that could be a sign of breast cancer. The doctor can tell a lot about a lump by carefully feeling it and the tissue around it. Benign lumps often feel different from cancerous ones.

11. What happens during a mammogram?

Mammography is a simple procedure. A registered technologist takes an x-ray of each breast with a machine that is used only for breast x-rays. It is different from x-ray machines that are used to take x-rays of the bones or other parts of the body. The standard mammogram exam includes two views of each breast, one from above and one angled from the side.

The technologist places the breast between two flat plastic plates. The two plates are then pressed together. The idea is to flatten the breast as much as possible. Spreading the tissue out makes any abnormal details easier to spot with a minimum of radiation. The technologist takes the x-ray, and then repeats the procedure for the next view. The pressure from the plates may be uncomfortable, or even slightly painful, but each x-ray takes less than one minute.

12. What are some of the possible benefits of a mammogram?

A mammogram can often detect breast changes in women who have no signs of breast cancer. Often, it can find a breast lump before it can be felt. If the results indicate that cancer might be present, your doctor will advise you to have a follow-up test called a biopsy.

13. How often should I have a mammogram?

Several studies show that mammography screening has reduced the number of deaths from breast cancer. However, some other studies have not shown a clear benefit from mammography. Scientists are continuing to examine the level of benefit that can come from mammography.

The National Cancer Institute recommends the following:

- If you are a woman in your 40s, you should have mammography screening every one to two years.
- If you are a woman age 50 and older, you should have mammography screening every one to two years.

- If you are a woman who is at higher than average risk for breast cancer, you should seek expert medical advice about whether to begin screening before age 40 and how often to have screening mammography.

14. Is there any danger in having a mammogram?

Some women worry about radiation exposure, but the risk of any harm from a mammogram is actually quite small. The doses of radiation used are very low and considered safe. The exact amount of radiation used during a mammogram will depend on several factors. For instance, breasts that are large or dense will require higher doses to get a clear image.

The federal government limits the amount of radiation used for each exposure of the breast to 0.3 rad. A "rad" is a unit of measurement that stands for Radiation Absorbed Dose. In practice, most mammograms deliver just a small fraction of this amount.

15. If a breast exam or mammogram does indicate the possibility of cancer, what happens next?

If the results of a clinical breast exam or a mammogram indicate that cancer might be present, the doctor will order a follow-up test. The most common follow-up test is called a biopsy. This is a procedure where a doctor removes a small amount of fluid or tissue from the breast to make a definitive diagnosis. A doctor might perform fine needle aspiration, a needle or "core" biopsy, or a surgical biopsy.

16. Are there other procedures being developed that might be better at diagnosing breast cancer?

Researchers have studied another type of surgical biopsy which removes less breast tissue. It is called an image-guided needle breast biopsy, or stereotactic biopsy. Eighty percent of U.S. women who have a surgical breast biopsy do not have cancer.

17. If I do need to seek treatment for breast cancer, what are some of my options?

You can seek conventional treatment from a specialized cancer doctor, called an oncologist. The oncologist will usually assemble a team of specialists to guide your therapy. Besides the oncologist, the team may include a surgeon, a radiation oncologist who is a specialist in radiation therapy, and others.

Before starting treatment, you may want another doctor to review the diagnosis and treatment plan. Some insurance companies require a second opinion. Others may pay for a second opinion if you request it. You might also be eligible to enroll in a clinical trial to receive treatment that conventional therapies may not offer.

18. What is a clinical trial and how do I know if it is right for me?

Clinical trials are research studies on people to find out whether a new drug or treatment is both safe and effective. New therapies are tested on people only after laboratory and animal studies show promising results. The Food and Drug Administration sets strict rules to make sure that people who agree to be in the studies are treated as safely as possible.

19. Before treatment begins, I have heard that the doctor will stage the cancer. What is staging?

Once breast cancer has been found, it is staged. Staging means determining how far the cancer has progressed. Through staging, the doctor can tell if the cancer has spread and, if so, to what parts of the body. More tests may be performed to help determine the stage. Knowing the stage of the disease helps the doctor plan treatment. Staging will let the doctor know

- the size of the tumor and exactly where it is in the breast.
- if the cancer has spread within the breast.
- if cancer is present in the lymph nodes under the arm.
- If cancer is present in other parts of the body.

20. What are the standard types of treatment for breast cancer?

Standard treatments for breast cancer include

- surgery that takes out the cancer
- radiation therapy that uses high-energy beams to kill cancer cells and shrink tumors
- chemotherapy that uses anti-cancer drugs to kill cancer cells
- hormone therapy that keeps cancer cells from getting the hormones they need to survive and grow.

21. What kinds of surgery are available for women with breast cancer?

Surgery, as opposed to chemotherapy or radiation, is the most common treatment for breast cancer. The kind of surgery a woman has is based on the type and stage of the cancer. Most women can choose between breast-conserving surgery that removes the cancer but not the breast, or surgery that removes the entire breast and sometimes the surrounding tissue.

22. What is involved in breast-conserving surgery?

There are two types of breast-conserving surgery -- lumpectomy and partial mastectomy.

- Lumpectomy is the removal of the tumor and a small amount of normal tissue around it. A woman who has a lumpectomy almost always has radiation therapy as well. Most surgeons also take out some of the lymph nodes under the arm.

- Partial or segmental mastectomy is removal of the cancer, some of the breast tissue around the tumor, and the lining over the chest muscles below the tumor. Often, surgeons remove some of the lymph nodes under the arm. In most cases, radiation therapy follows.

23. What does a mastectomy involve?

Surgery to remove the entire breast and sometimes the surrounding tissue is called a mastectomy. There are three types:

- A total or simple mastectomy is removal of the whole breast. Sometimes the surgeon takes out lymph nodes under the arm as well.

- A modified radical mastectomy is removal of the breast, many of the lymph nodes under the arm, and the lining over the chest muscles. Sometimes, the surgeon removes part of the chest wall muscles, too.

- A radical mastectomy, sometimes called the Halsted radical mastectomy, is removal of the breast, chest muscles, and all of the lymph nodes under the arm. This surgery is used only when the tumor has spread to the chest muscles.

24. Are there any treatments that follow surgery?

Even if the surgeon removes all of the cancer that can be seen at the time of surgery, a woman may still receive follow-up treatment. This may include radiation therapy, chemotherapy, or hormone therapy to try to kill any cancer cells that may be left. Treatment that a patient receives after surgery to increase the chances of a cure is called adjuvant therapy.

25. How and when is breast reconstruction done?

Breast reconstruction, surgery to rebuild a breast's shape, is often an option after mastectomy. Some health insurance plans pay for all or part of the cost of breast reconstruction. Often, they will pay for surgery to the other breast so that both breasts are about the same shape and size.

If you are thinking about reconstruction, you should talk with a plastic surgeon before your mastectomy. Some women begin reconstruction at the same time as they have the mastectomy done. Others wait several months or even years. Although the reconstructed breast will not have natural sensation, the surgery can give you a result that looks like a breast.

The reconstructed breast may be made with the patient's own, non-breast tissue or by using implants filled with saline or silicone gel. The Food and Drug Administration has decided that breast implants filled with silicone gel may be used only in clinical trials. Before making the decision to get an implant, a woman can call the Food and Drug Administration's Center for Devices and Radiologic Health at 1-888-INFO-FDA or 1-888-463-6332 for more information.

26. How is radiation therapy used to treat breast cancer?
Radiation therapy uses high-energy x-rays or other types of radiation to kill cancer cells and shrink tumors. This therapy often follows a lumpectomy, and is sometimes used after mastectomy. During radiation therapy, a machine outside the body sends high-energy beams to kill the cancer cells that may still be present in the affected breast or in nearby lymph nodes. Doctors sometimes use radiation therapy along with chemotherapy, or before or instead of surgery.

27. How is chemotherapy used to treat breast cancer?
Chemotherapy is the use of drugs to kill cancer cells. A patient may take chemotherapy by mouth in pill form, or it may be put into the body by inserting a needle into a vein or muscle. Chemotherapy is called whole body or systemic

treatment if the drugs enter the bloodstream, travel through the body, and can kill cancer cells throughout the body. Treatment with standard chemotherapy can be as short as two months or as long as two years. In this decade, targeted therapies, usually in pill form, have become more common and focus on either a gene or protein abnormality and usually have few adverse side-effects.

Sometimes chemotherapy is the only treatment the doctor will recommend. More often, however, chemotherapy is used in addition to surgery, radiation therapy, and/or biological therapy.

28. How is hormonal therapy used to treat breast cancer?

Hormonal therapy keeps cancer cells from getting the hormones they need to grow. This treatment may include the use of drugs that change the way hormones work. Sometimes it includes surgery to remove the ovaries, which make female hormones. Like chemotherapy, hormonal therapy can affect cancer cells throughout the body.

Often, women with early-stage breast cancer and those with metastatic breast cancer -- meaning cancer that has spread to other parts of the body -- receive hormone therapy in the form of tamoxifen. Hormone therapy with tamoxifen or estrogens can act on cells all over the body. However, it may increase the chance of developing endometrial cancer. If you take tamoxifen, you should have a pelvic examination every year to look for any signs of cancer. A woman should report any vaginal bleeding, other than menstrual bleeding, to her doctor as soon as possible.

29. What drugs are available?

Certain drugs that have been used successfully in other cancers are now being used to treat some breast cancers. A mix of drugs may increase the length of time you will live, or the length of time you will live without cancer.

In addition, certain drugs like Herceptin® and Tykerb® taken in combination with chemotherapy, can help women with specific genetic breast cancer mutations better than chemotherapy alone.

30. What is the best way to prevent breast cancer?

Several methods can reduce breast cancer risk. Following a large-scale study, researchers found that tamoxifen reduced cancer in high-risk women by about 50 percent.

Another method is a type of surgery called preventive or prophylactic mastectomy for women at high risk of breast cancer. It involves removing a breast that is not known to contain cancer in order to reduce a woman's cancer risk.

31. What is the relationship between lifestyle and breast cancer?

Some researchers are looking at diet as a possible risk factor for breast cancer. Studies show that women in populations that consume a high-fat diet are more likely to die of breast cancer than women in populations that consume a low fat diet. But scientists still do not know for sure if a diet low in fat will lower the risk of breast cancer, or if any other specific dietary changes will actually prevent cancer.

Some studies point to lifestyle choices that may decrease a woman's risk of breast cancer. Exercise, especially in young women, may decrease hormone levels and contribute to a decreased risk. Breast-feeding also may decrease risk.

Other studies point to lifestyle factors that might increase a woman's risk of developing breast cancer. For instance, women who drink alcohol have a slightly increased risk. Gaining weight after menopause, especially after natural menopause and/or after age 60, also may increase a woman's risk.

32. Are there new studies under way to try and reduce a woman's chance of getting breast cancer?

Research shows women with early-stage breast cancer who took the drug letrozole, an aromatase inhibitor, after they completed five years of tamoxifen therapy significantly reduced their risk of breast cancer recurrence.

Also, other research found a test that can predict both the risk of breast cancer recurrence and who is most likely to benefit from chemotherapy such as letrozole.

Another study, known as TAILORx, was launched by the National Cancer Institute to examine whether genes that are frequently associated with risk of recurrence for women with early-stage breast cancer can be used to assign patients to the most appropriate and effective treatment.

33. Are there other options for someone with breast cancer?

Some breast cancer patients take part in studies of new treatments. These studies -- called clinical trials -- are designed to find out whether a new treatment is both safe and effective. Often, clinical trials compare a new treatment with a standard one so that doctors can learn which is more effective. People with breast cancer who are interested in taking part in a clinical trial should talk with their doctor.

34. Where can I find a comprehensive analysis of research on breast cancer?

The National Cancer Institute has developed a comprehensive online cancer database called the Physician Data Query, or PDQ, to present evidence on the most recent research on breast cancer.

www.MedicalCenter.com

www.ingramcontent.com/pod-product-compliance
Lightning Source LLC
Chambersburg PA
CBHW071547170526
45166CB00004B/1574